Lose 50 pounds and keep the weight off without exercising!

By Dave Lack

TITLE: Lose 50 pounds and keep the weight off without exercising!

<u>Introduction:</u>

Whether you want to lose five pounds or 100 pounds, you can use my techniques to meet your weight loss goals. I lost more than 50 pounds and you can too! When you follow my eating plans, you will lose and maintain your weight. Real success is not only losing the weight but keeping the weight off.

By teaching you to eat healthier, setting a calorie limit each day, letting you decide how much weight to lose each week and giving you permission to eat the foods you crave, **you** personalize your own weight loss journey. I will also share my journey with you.

If you are like me you've battled with what to eat most of your life. You know you should eat healthier. Deep down inside, you knew you were making bad decisions. My eating plans will guide you and help you make the right decisions. Success isn't always a straight upward line. If you stumble, I show you how to get back on your weight loss journey. People keep asking, "how did you lose your weight?"

I decided to share what worked for me. I hope you find it useful.

Questions about this plan

Can you lose 50 pounds and keep the weight off? Absolutely!

Will it be difficult? Not as hard as you think.

Is this a diet? No this is an eating plan. You will change your relationship with food.

What are the two main benefits of your eating plan? My plan trains you to eat healthier and allows you to earn the right to eat whatever you want when you are under your weekly goal.

Why is allowing me the ability to eat whatever I want so important? Because the biggest problem with a diet is that people do not have the will power to completely give up their favorite foods.

Who are you? My name is Dave Lack and I recently lost more than 50 pounds. I live in Southern California, I am 58 years old and I'm 5'10". I decided to write this book because people kept asking me, "How did you lose your weight?" I used to weigh 238 pounds and I now weigh 178 pounds. This plan will work for any weight loss goal.

Are you a doctor, dietician, nurse or any other medical professional? No, I am not. I do not have any medical training whatsoever. You should never change your eating habits without consulting a medical expert. I am simply detailing how I lost and kept my weight off.

How much do I need to spend to be on this eating plan? All you need is a digital scale to weigh yourself.

What's the most important thing I need to do to be successful on this plan? You need to weigh yourself every morning when you are at home.

How fast can I lose the weight? That's up to you. This is not a plan that is geared for a quick loss of weight. This approach changes your eating habits allowing you to keep the weight off. If you need to lose 50 pounds in six weeks, this plan is not for you.

What do you have against exercise? I don't have anything against exercise. Personally, I couldn't both change what I ate and start exercising more often. If you can do both at the same time, then go ahead. I am active but I'm not the kind of guy who is going to have a daily exercise routine.

<u>My weight loss journey</u>

I didn't think about my weight every day. In fact, I rarely thought about my weight. I knew I wasn't skinny but I didn't think I was obese. Most days I walked past the bathroom scale. I looked in the mirror to shave, not noticing my weight.

I would look at pictures from special occasions or vacations. I looked a little heavy, not obese, just heavy. My heaviest weight was 238 pounds. I am 5' 10". I used to be 5' 11" but I lost an inch somewhere. No jokes please. Sometimes after looking at the pictures, I would decide to diet. I remember doing a diet with cabbage soup. You had to make the soup yourself, store the soup in the refrigerator and then eat the soup two or three times a day. Looking back, that was crazy. Every week for the rest of your life you make cabbage soup and eat it two or three times a day. What kind of plan is that?

I went on the all meat diet once. What I remember about this diet is it was no carbs, just meat. I'm sure there is more to it, but that's what comes to mind now. I think it worked for a while. I lost some weight, I think my breath stunk and I missed pasta. I like pasta. I couldn't do this all meat thing forever.

Sometimes people would make comments about my weight or my meal portions. Comments like "hey big guy", "boy you really like that fried chicken" or a suit tailor pointing at my stomach saying "do you have any plans about this". Those comments stung. Later, I would think if you want to stop the comments you should lose some weight.

I was getting older and I decided I should start getting annual physicals. I don't like going to the doctor. The first three physicals basically went the same. I was borderline unhealthy on pretty much every test. My doctor would say he would like me to eat healthier and try to lose some weight. I would go home with good intentions. I would eat healthier for a while then I would fall back into my old habits. I often wonder why I didn't do better. I would exaggerate to myself the good things I did, but the unhealthy things I just continued to do. If I ordered a salad at lunch or had less to eat at dinner I would feel good. What I didn't change were all the bad habits. I kept drinking beers at happy hour and ordering fried food. I would have too many servings at dinner and eat late at night. The weight stayed with me.

In June of 2015 after my physical, my doctor told me my cardiac risk was above average. This news got my attention. My Uncle Joe had died early of a heart condition. He was overweight. I always have considered him my guardian angel. Many years after he had died, he whispered in my ear, "You will marry that women" when I first saw my wife, (that's another book). My doctor wanted me to lose weight and change my diet; he would refer me to a nutritionist if I desired. I declined his offer and thought, I can lose the weight. This time I was committed; thanks, Uncle Joe.

Ready, Set, Diet! I was mentally ready. I bought salads to work for lunch. I bought low sugar cereal to eat for breakfast and for dinner I was going to have smaller portions. I put a calorie app on my phone and recorded everything I was eating. I was losing weight and I felt good. I did this for a month and I was down about ten pounds. I weighed somewhere around 225 pounds. I wasn't sure what my weight should be. I figured if I could get under 200 pounds that would be great. I looked at the BMI (body mass index) and for a 5' 10" man, the recommended normal weight was under 173 pounds. I didn't like that. There was no way I was going to weigh 173 pounds. I was happy with my weight loss but I was craving the foods I wasn't eating (fries, burgers, pizza) and I lost my momentum. I started to slip back into my old eating habits and in two weeks I had gained back five of the ten pounds I had lost. That's when I said to myself, you need to come up with a plan or you are going to gain the weight back.

I asked myself, "What's the easiest goal I can achieve?" I decided to make it easy and simply try to lose ½ pound or a pound a week (you can be more aggressive than I was, more on that later). If I only lost ½ pound a week, I would be 26 pounds lighter in one year!

That's how my path to losing more than 50 pounds started. What I didn't realize at the time is that losing weight slowly and consistently would teach me how to maintain my weight once I reached my desired weight. Now look in the mirror and tell yourself you can lose ½ pound a week.

<u>It's time for you to lose weight and keep the weight off!</u>

Let me help you. My eating plans will guide you on how many calories to eat each day based on your daily weight and your weekly goals. With any change, you might feel uneasy at first but if you stick with it you will become more comfortable. If you fail one day, don't give up! The next day just go back to the eating plan recommendations. Success isn't always a straight upward line. Good luck and stay the course as best you can.

Let's get started!

First some definitions of terms we will be using. There is a 30-day example later in the book that will clarify these terms.

Starting weight: This is your weight on the first day when you decide to start following the eating plans.

Daily Weight: This is your weight when you weigh yourself in the morning.

Weekly Goal: Each week you will decide how much weight you want to lose. Your weekly weight loss goal can be as little as a half-pound a week to three pounds a week. I wouldn't be any more aggressive than three pounds a week. You can change the number of pounds you want to lose each week but you must always commit to losing weight each week. Your weekly goal must be lower each week even if you did not meet your goal from the previous week. Continue with this weekly process until you have reached your desired weight. Please see the 30-day example later in the book to understand how to set your weekly goal.

Over/under goal: The difference between your daily weight and your weekly goal will determine which eating plan you follow for that day.

Desired Maintenance Weight: Decide what weight you want to maintain. What weight will make you happy? Deciding what weight, you want to maintain is different than saying how much weight do you want to lose. Declaring, "I want to lose 50 pounds" doesn't prepare you for keeping the weight off. The goal is to maintain your weight. Too many times, people lose the weight and then gain it back. This will not happen to you if you follow the eating plans. Real success is not only losing the weight but keeping the weight off. You can do it!

__Eating plans__

There are five eating plans that will dictate what you can eat each day. Every morning you weigh yourself. You compare your daily weight to your weekly goal. The difference in pounds between your daily weight and your weekly goal will determine what you eat that day. Once you have reached your desired weight, continue to use the eating plan guidelines to maintain your weight. This plan will change your eating habits, improve your health and make sure you keep the weight off.

The eating plans are listed below. For now, just read through them and look at the eating plan breakdown. We will go through an example after you familiarize yourself with the eating plans.

Eating Plan #1- *__Your weight is more than two pounds over your weekly goal.__*

Eat a breakfast under 200 calories, a lunch under 350 calories and a dinner under 650 calories. You are allowed one 100 calorie or lower snack and unlimited fruit and vegetables. No desserts.

Eating Plan #2- _Your weight is over your weekly goal by two pounds or less._

Eat a breakfast under 200 calories, a lunch under 350 calories and a dinner under 900 calories. You are allowed one 100 calorie or lower snack and unlimited fruit and vegetables. No desserts.

Eating Plan #3 - _Your weight is at your weekly goal or lower than your goal by two pounds or less._

Eat a breakfast under 200 calories, a lunch under 350 calories and for dinner you can eat anything you desire. You must eat dinner before 8 p.m. If you eat dinner after 8 p.m., then dinner can only be 650 calories. You are allowed one 100 calorie or lower snack and unlimited fruit and vegetables. You are also allowed one dessert under 400 calories.

Eating Plan #4- _Your weight is under your weekly goal between 2.1 to four pounds._

Eat one low calorie meal a day (either breakfast under 200 calories, lunch under 350 calories or dinner under 900 calories). The other two meals you can eat whatever you want. You are allowed one 100 calorie or lower snack and unlimited fruit and vegetables. Dinner must be before 8 p.m. If you eat dinner after 8 p.m., then dinner can only be 650 calories. You are also allowed one dessert under 700 calories.

Eating plan #5- ***Your weight is four pounds or more under your goal***

Enjoy your success and eat anything you desire! Eat anytime of the day!

Counting Calories: Eating plans #1 through #4 involve counting calories. There are many phone applications you can use for counting calories. You can also find calorie information on nutrition labels. Make sure you look at calorie counts per serving size. Many restaurants now put calorie counts on their menus.

Eating plan breakdown below

Google Doc link for home printing of table: https://tinyurl.com/ycopb34o

Eating plans	Eating Plan #1	Eating Plan #2	Eating Plan #3	Eating Plan #4	Eating Plan #5
Your weight today	is more than two pounds over your weekly goal.	is over your weekly goal by two pounds or less	is at your weekly goal or lower than your goal by two pounds or less	is under your weekly goal between 2.1 to four pounds	is four pounds or more under your weekly goal
Breakfast	200 calories or less	200 calories or less	200 calories or less	one low calorie meal a day, other meals eat what you want	eat what you want
Lunch	350 calories or less	350 calories or less	350 calories or less	one low calorie meal a day, other meals eat what you want	eat what you want
Dinner before 8pm	650 calories or less	900 calories or less	eat what you want	one low calorie meal a day, other meals eat what you want	eat what you want
Dessert	no dessert	no dessert	any dessert under 400 calories	any dessert under 700 calories	eat what you want
Snack	100 calories or less	100 calories or less	100 calories or less	100 calories or less	eat what you want
Vegetables	eat what you want	eat what you want	eat what you want	eat what you want	eat what you want
Fruit	eat what you want	eat what you want	eat what you want	eat what you want	eat what you want

* all dinners in Eating plans one through four must be eaten by 8pm. If after 8 pm dinner, must be under 650 calories. Note # : You may substitute calorie counts between meals. For example if you are in Eating plan two and you want to have a breakfast of 900 calories you can do that but your dinner will need to be 200 calories or less. Google Doc link for home printing of table: https://tinyurl.com/y7ulwhsw

Let's look at a 30-day example for losing weight

Day 1:

Jenny has decided that she wants to lose a pound a week. She weighs 200 pounds this morning- this will be her starting weight. By next Monday, she needs to weigh 199 pounds. As she weighs 200 pounds and her goal is to be at 199 pounds, she is one pound over her goal weight for the week. For today she will follow Eating Plan #2. ***Eating Plan #2 is designed for days where your weight is over your weekly goal by two pounds or less.***

Day 2:

Jenny weighs herself Tuesday morning and she weighs 199.5 pounds. Her goal is 199 pounds so she is a half- pound over her goal. She will follow Eating Plan #2 again today.

Day 3:

Jenny weighs herself Wednesday morning. She weighs 199 pounds. Her weekly goal is 199 pounds. She is at her goal so she will follow ***Eating Plan # 3 as her weight is at her weekly goal or lower than her goal by two pounds or less.***

Day 4:

Jenny weighs herself Thursday morning and she
weighs 198.5 pounds. Her weekly goal is 199
pounds. Since she is a half-pound under her goal
she will follow Eating Plan #3 again today.

Day 5:

Jenny weighs herself Friday morning and she
weighs 198 pounds. Her weekly goal is 199
pounds. Since she is one pound under her goal
she will follow Eating Plan #3 today.

Day 6:

Jenny weighs herself Saturday morning and she
weighs 199.5 pounds. Jenny went out for happy
hour after work on Friday and had a few drinks
and some appetizers. She also had a piece of
cheesecake. Her weekly goal is 199 pounds.
She will follow Eating Plan #2 today as she
is half a pound over her goal. ***Eating Plan #2
is adhered to when your weight is over your
weekly goal by two pounds or less.***

Day 7:

Jenny weighs herself Sunday morning and
she weighs 199.5 pounds, the same weight as
Saturday. Her weekly goal is 199

pounds. She will follow Eating Plan #2 again today

Day 8 - New Week:

Jenny weighs herself Monday morning and she weighs 199 pounds. This is a new week. She is happy she met last week's goal of 199 pounds. Since today starts a new week, Jenny has decided to lower her weekly goal by one pound this week. Her new goal this week will be 198 pounds. She is one pound over her weekly goal of 198 pounds so today she will follow Eating Plan # 2.

Day 9:

Jenny weighs herself Tuesday morning and she weighs 198.5 pounds. Her goal is 198 pounds so she is a half- pound over her goal. She will follow Eating Plan #2 today.

Day 10:

Jenny weighs herself Wednesday morning. She weighs 198 pounds. Her weekly goal is 198 pounds. She is at her goal so she will follow ***Eating Plan # 3 as her weight is at her weekly goal or lower than her goal by two pounds or less.***

Day 11:

Jenny weighs herself Thursday morning and she weighs 199 pounds. Her weekly goal is 198 pounds. Jenny had a late-night dinner after 8pm. She was at a restaurant and she tried to stay on her eating plan but she is not sure she did because there were no calorie counts on the menu. Since she is a pound over her goal she will follow Eating Plan #2 today. ***Eating Plan #2 is followed when your weight is over your weekly goal by two pounds or less***.

Day 12:

Jenny had a big project at work Friday morning and forgot to weigh herself. Since she followed eating plan #2 on Day 11, so she will follow eating plan #2 again today.

Day 13:

Jenny weighs herself Saturday morning and she weighs 199 pounds. Her weekly goal is 198 pounds. She will follow Eating Plan #2 today because she is a pound over her goal.

Day 14:

Jenny weighs herself Sunday morning and she weighs 200.5 pounds. She went to a party Saturday night and went "way off my eating plan." Her weekly goal is 198 pounds. Today she will follow ***Eating Plan #1 because her weight is more than two pounds over her goal.***

Day 15 - New Week:

Jenny weighs herself Monday morning and she weighs 199.5 pounds. This is a new week. She is disappointed she did not meet last week's goal of 198 pounds. Since today starts a new week Jenny has decided that she only wants to try and lower her weekly goal by half a pound this week. Last week her goal was 198 pounds, this week she only wants to lower the goal by a half a pound so her weekly goal this week will be 197.5 pounds. She is two pounds over her weekly goal of 197.5 pounds so today she will follow Eating Plan # 2. ***Eating Plan #2 is followed to when your weight is over your weekly goal by two pounds or less.***

Day 16:

Jenny weighs herself Tuesday morning and she weighs 198.5 pounds. Her weekly goal is 197.5 pounds so she is a pound over her goal. She will follow Eating Plan #2 today.

Day 17:

Jenny weighs herself Wednesday morning. She weighs 197.5 pounds. Her weekly goal is

197.5 pounds. She is at her goal so today she will follow ***Eating Plan # 3 as her weight is at her weekly goal or lower than her goal by two pounds or less.***

Day 18:

Jenny weighs herself Thursday morning and she weighs 197 pounds. Her weekly goal is 197.5 pounds. Since she is a half-pound under her goal she will follow Eating Plan #3 today.

Day 19:

Jenny weighs herself Friday Morning and she weighs 196 pounds. Her weekly goal is 197.5 pounds. Since she is one and a half pounds under her goal she will follow Eating Plan #3 today.

Day 20:

Jenny weighs herself Saturday morning and she weighs 195.5 pounds. Her weekly goal is 197.5 pounds. She will follow Eating Plan #3 today because she is two pounds under her goal.

Day 21:

Jenny weighs herself Sunday Morning and weighs 195.3 pounds. Her weekly goal is 197.5 pounds. Jenny is 2.2 pounds under her weekly goal. She will follow ***Eating Plan #4 today as her weight is under her weekly goal between 2.1 to four pounds.***

Day 22 – New Week:

Jenny weighs herself Monday morning and she weighs 196 pounds. This is a new week, she is happy she met last week's goal of 197.5 pounds. Jenny has decided to lower her weekly goal by a half a pound this week. Her new goal this week is 197 pounds. She is one pound under her weekly goal of 197 pounds so today she will follow Eating Plan # 3. ***Eating Plan #3 is adhered to when your weight is at your weekly goal or lower than her goal by two pounds or less.***

Day 23:

Jenny weighs herself Tuesday morning and she weighs 195.2 pounds. Her weekly goal is 197 pounds. She is 1.8 pounds under her goal. She will follow Eating Plan #3 today.

Day 24:

Jenny weighs herself Wednesday morning. She weighs 194 pounds. Her weekly goal is 197 pounds. She is three pounds under her goal so today she will follow Eating Plan # 4. ***Eating Plan #4 is adhered to when your weight is***

<u>under your weekly goal between 2.1 to four pounds.</u>

Day 25:

Jenny weighs herself Thursday morning and she weighs 193 pounds. Her weekly goal is 197 pounds. Since she is four pounds under her goal she will follow Eating Plan #4 today.

Day 26:

Jenny weighs herself Friday morning and she weighs 192.8 pounds. Her weekly goal is 197 pounds. Since she is 4.2 pounds under her goal she will follow ***<u>Eating Plan #5 today because her weight is four pounds or more under her goal. She gets to eat anything she wants!</u>***

Day 27:

Jenny weighs herself Saturday morning and she weighs 194 pounds. Her weekly goal is 197 pounds. She will follow Eating Plan #4 today because she is three pounds under her goal. ***<u>Eating Plan #4 is adhered to when your weight is under your weekly goal between 2.1 to four pounds.</u>***

Day 28:

Jenny weighs herself Sunday morning and she weighs 194.4 pounds. Her weekly goal is 197 pounds. Jenny is 2.6 pounds under her weekly goal. She will follow Eating Plan #4 today.

Day 29 – New Week:

Jenny weighs herself Monday morning and she weighs 195 pounds. This is a new week, she is happy she met last week's goal of 197 pounds. Jenny has decided to lower her weekly goal by a pound this week. Her new goal this week is 196 pounds. She is one pound under her weekly goal of 196 pounds so today she will follow Eating Plan # 3. ___**Eating Plan #3 is adhered to when your weight is at your weekly goal or lower than her goal by two pounds or less.**___

Day 30:

Jenny weighs herself Tuesday morning and she weighs 195.2 pounds. Her weekly goal is 196 pounds. She is .8 pounds under her goal. She will follow eating plan #3 today.

Wow, that example was tedious reading. Thanks for sticking with it!

<u>Recap</u>

You continue to use the appropriate eating plan every day. You continue to lower your weekly goal until you have reached your desired weight.

Once you have reached your desired weight, you continue to weigh yourself each day. You continue to use the eating plan that corresponds to the weight difference between your desired weight and what you weigh each day.

In the back of the book there are more eating plan examples. One example details how you maintain your desired weight and another example details eating tips you can use while traveling.

<u>Eating Plan Questions</u>

Can I have more calories at breakfast or lunch and less calories at dinner? Yes, you can. If you want to have a big lunch, then flip flop your dinner calories with your lunch calories. You can do the same with breakfast. The key is to keep your total calories for the day the same.

Can I have less calories at breakfast or lunch and more calories at dinner? Yes, you can but you cannot skip breakfast or lunch entirely. For example, if you have 300 calories at lunch instead of 350 calories then yes you can add 50 calories to dinner. The same goes for breakfast.

What you cannot to do is go the whole day without eating, saving your calories for dinner.

Do I need to eat at least three times a day? It is preferred that you eat three meals a day. If you skip a meal make sure you don't get light headed. For me, if I skip a meal, I have less control when I do eat. I would check with a medical expert before you decide to skip meals on a regular basis.

In the beginning is it easier to lose weight? When you first start your eating plan, you will lose weight faster. Remember my eating plan is geared toward keeping the weight off. If you want a slow steady loss of weight, you can start your eating plan with the goal of losing a half pound a week. If you want to lose weight faster, you can be more aggressive with your weekly goals. Instead of having a goal to lose half a pound a week make your goal something more aggressive like losing a pound or two pounds a week. I had the will power to be more aggressive in the beginning of my eating plan but after about six weeks I found myself slipping back into unhealthy habits. I think this will happen to most people. When this occurs, reset your goal to losing a half a pound a week. I think the goal of losing a half a pound a week is something most people can challenge themselves to do.

Can I stop before I reach my maintenance weight goal? Sure, you can but the key is not to slide back into a heavier weight. So, if you stop, use the eating plans to maintain your weight. You will continue to weigh yourself each day. You will compare your daily weight to the stopped weight. Do not gain the weight back!

Why does this plan have a better chance of working then other eating plans? There are two main reasons, one is you are monitoring your weight every day and adjusting you're eating habits accordingly. Two, you are learning to eat healthier.

When does the eating, plan result in a healthier life style? The eating plans train you to eat healthier and changes your expectations of what you will and can eat. If you follow the eating plans, you will be managing your weight, resulting in a healthier lifestyle. My food cravings have expanded. Before the eating plan, I would crave cheeseburgers, fries, tater tots, pizza, chicken wings, pasta, fried chicken and other fried and fatty foods. I am now beginning to crave some healthy foods. I crave salmon, seabass, avocado sandwich, apple slices, chicken noodle soup, pineapple, strawberries, Brussels sprouts and other healthier choices. I crave healthy foods now!

Can I cheat a little? Yes, you can. Let's say you are at dinner and the table orders a dessert. Go ahead and take one bite, it won't ruin your eating plan. One bite of anything is fine.

Another cheat is to pick one food item that you love but is not available to you every day or every week. My item is freshly made kettle corn. If I am at a festival, fair or local baseball game and someone is making fresh kettle corn, I can have some.

How do I adjust my eating plan based on where and when I eat?

When to eat: Having dinner past 8 p.m. is a bad idea. If you find yourself eating dinner past 8 p.m., make it a healthy dinner and keep the calories below 650. Pick fish or a healthy entrée salad. Breakfast and lunch, try to eat around the same time each day.

Can I eat what my family is having for dinner or do I need to eat something different:
I encourage you to eat what your family is having for dinner, just watch the portions. You can usually use a calorie counting app to get a rough idea of how many calories your meal will contain. If you miscalculate by a couple of calories it's okay, family dinner time is worth it. Do not criticize the rest of the family about their eating habits, just follow your eating plan guidelines. If someone in your family sees your weight loss and they are motivated to lose weight, they will ask you, "How are you losing the weight?" You can then share your plan with them. If your family always has fried foods or fatty foods, then try to bring in some healthier foods or add some vegetables and fruits to the meals.

Holiday Pass Days, you can eat whatever you want! I believe in making the holidays special and that includes eating whatever you want. On these holidays, you can eat whatever you want: New Year's Eve, New Year's Day, Easter (religious equivalent if not Christian), Memorial Day, July Fourth, Labor Day, Thanksgiving, Christmas (substitute another religious holiday if not Christian), and your birthday. That's nine days out of the year you can eat whatever you want! Enjoy these days, make them special. Sorry, no calorie splurging on minor holidays like sweetest day or national cheeseburger day.

Eating at restaurants: Most restaurants will have a low-calorie section of the menu and you should select items from this section. If you are in a restaurant where the calories are listed by each food item, then simply pick a food item that meets your calorie requirements. If you are at a restaurant that does not have a low- calorie menu or does not list the number of calories by each menu item then you should use the eating guidelines for salad, soup, fish or chicken (see below) when you place your order. Going to restaurants is enjoyable and I would never tell you not to dine out. Eating at home is preferred though because you can control your calorie intake and you are less tempted to go off your eating plan.

Eating at home: Eating at home gives you the most control over your food choices. You can plan your meals and home meals are generally less expensive. Keep the high-calorie tempting foods out of your house.

Travel: I think the hardest time to stay on an eating plan is when you travel, especially if you are drinking alcohol on your trip. Airport food, client dinners, office parties, all night work sessions, meals with friends, late night parties and feeling less restrained all contribute to poor eating habits. These play havoc with an eating plan. You need to prepare yourself!

I don't find it practical to carry a scale around with me when I travel. If you want to carry a scale along when you travel, go ahead, it won't hurt and it may be what you need to make sure you continue to weigh yourself each day. If you carry a scale with you, then just follow the eating plan requirements as you do when you are home.

When I travel (assuming I am in eating plan one through four), I allow myself one bad meal every three days on the trip. I don't always give in to having one bad meal but if I do, I don't beat myself up over it. The other days I follow the eating guidelines in the eating plan I am in when I leave for the trip. The most important thing to remember is when you get back from your trip, weigh yourself at home the next morning and every morning you are at home. If you are in Eating Plan # 5 you can eat whatever you want but remember you need to weigh yourself when you get back home. If you are no longer in Eating Plan # 5 when you get home, you need to adjust accordingly. See the travel eating plan example at the end of the book.

Parties: Adhering to your eating plan at parties is difficult. I think you should have a good time and keep the calories low. If food is offered avoid the same type of foods, you would avoid at a restaurant. Snack on shrimp cocktail, salads, pretzels and fruit. Alcohol is discussed below.

 Breakfast: I usually have an English muffin with a little bit of butter. An English muffin is around 150 calories, the butter adds another 50 calories. You can also have fruit, oatmeal or a low-calorie breakfast bar.

Lunch: I usually have a fresh salad that is under 300 calories. The salads are healthy and they are inexpensive. You can buy low-calorie frozen entrees. If you go out for lunch stick to salads (see below), fruit, sashimi, grilled chicken and soup.

Dinner: Grilled chicken, grilled pork chops, fresh baked or grilled fish should be your main proteins. Pair it with vegetables, fruit, rice and salad.

Of course, if you are in Eating Plan # 5 you can eat whatever you want!

Guidelines for specific food categories:

Salads: All salads are not low calorie. Stay away from salads containing anything fried, bacon, taco shells, lots of cheese or heavy cream or barbequed type dressings. Choose a low-calorie dressing, balsamic vinegar dressing or a low-fat dressing. If you want, request the dressing on the side. Grilled chicken or fish in a salad is OK. Stay away from taco salads and Greek salads as they are usually very high in calories.

Soups: Clear broth is better than cream broth. Soup with vegetables, chicken and fish are best. Tomato based soups are fine. Stay away from cream based broths.

Fish: Any grilled or blackened fish is fine. Do not eat fish that is crusted with any sort of nut or breading. Do not eat fried fish of any kind. Grilled shrimp and scallops also work but make sure they are not coated in butter. No fried shrimp. Have your grilled fish with rice or fruit. Avoid fish sandwiches or fish tacos (if you get fish tacos, soft corn tortilla tacos are best), the bread adds on calories.

Sushi and Sashimi: I love sushi and sashimi. You can eat as much sashimi as you like. Sushi has more calories because of the rice. Your basic sushi is ok, it's the rolls that can get you in trouble. Don't order sushi rolls with anything fried or with cream cheese. Stay away from rolls with any type of mayonnaise.

Chicken: Grilled chicken breast (skinless) is the best choice. Fried chicken is not a good option. You can top your grilled chicken with vegetables or some type of salsa. Limit the cheese.

Turkey: Turkey breast is a good option. Watch the gravy. Skinless is best.

Pork: A lean grilled pork chop is good. I love ribs but the BBQ sauce can have a lot of sugar or molasses and the ribs themselves have higher calories than a lean pork chop.

Red Meat: I prefer white meat over red meat but some red meat is low in calories. A filet mignon or a lean cut of beef often has low calories. The more fat on the meat usually means more calories, so stay away from rib eye and other fatty cuts. Watch the sauces on your steak, basic seasoning is best. Lamb is usually high in calories.

Snacks: Buy your snacks in the 100 calorie bags. If you cannot buy the 100 calorie bags, then count out your snacks before you eat them. For example, I know one Pringle chip is about ten calories. I don't sit down and start eating from the large Pringle can and count to ten chips then try to stop. I know that is too difficult for me. What I will do is count out ten chips, put the large can back in the pantry and eat just the ten chips I counted out. This process works because you will need to make an additional effort to eat more than ten chips.

If you want to substitute a food item you are really craving as your snack you can do it but you cannot eat more than 100 calories of this item. I personally do not have the will power to do this. If you find yourself cheating on the snacks, only eat snacks you know you have the will power to handle.

Fruit and vegetables: The big issue for me is how do avoid wasting fresh fruits and vegetables. Buy a whole cantaloupe or watermelon and cut it up and store it in a container. The small bags of sliced apples are a good snack. The no- sugar- added mandarin orange containers that kids use for their lunches is a good choice. I like the frozen single packet edamame containers you heat up in the microwave. The small packages of baby carrots are a good vegetable choice. Low calorie or no calorie pickles are also something you can store in the refrigerator for a long time. Remember, on this eating plan you can have unlimited amounts of fruit and vegetables.

Processed Sugar: I am not a fan of processed sugar. I try to maintain a ratio of three grams of carbohydrates to one gram of processed sugar. Natural sugar is fine and items with no added sugar are fine, but it is the processed sugar that is troublesome. So, for example when I order girl scout cookies, I always look at the nutritional information. Usually I can just get the shortbread cookies but some years they have the peanut butter sandwich cookies I can order. Use the nutrition label on foods you buy to gauge the sugar to carbohydrate ratio.

Desserts: As I mentioned above, I don't do processed sugar unless the ratio is equal to or greater than three grams carbohydrates to one gram of sugar. There are a lot of no-sugar-added desserts out there, I like the no- sugar- added Klondike Bars and no- sugar- added ice cream. I am not a big fan of sugar-free items just because I don't like the taste but if you are OK with the taste go for it. Remember just because it's no-sugar-added or a sugar-free dessert does not mean it is low in calories. Always check.

Alcohol: I enjoy an adult beverage from time to time. How do you keep your calories low if you are drinking? I will drink vodka, club soda with a lime. A shot of vodka is around 90 calories, club soda has zero calories and a squeeze of lime adds some no calorie flavor. You can have most non-cream based liquors with club soda, diet tonic or diet soda and be OK calorie wise. Avoid beer if you can; I gain a lot of weight even if I drink light beers. A glass of wine has about 125 calories. Generally white wine has fewer calories than red wine. **Caution:** when you order mixed drinks, the alcohol content is more unpredictable than a beer so be careful of your intake. When you drink, you will also be more likely to go off your eating plan. If you want a margarita when you are in Mexico or at a Mexican restaurant go ahead and get one or two; it won't ruin your eating plan, just don't do it too often.

Non-alcoholic drinks: I am not a fan of soda. I almost always drink water, coffee or tea. If I am tired, I sometimes will drink a can of no sugar Red Bull. I hear mixed things about diet sodas and their effects on weight. I keep it simple, I don't drink soda of any kind unless I am mixing a diet soda or club soda with alcohol.

Fried Food: The bottom line is fried food has lots of calories and it's not healthy for you. Substitute fries with steamed vegetables or tomatoes.

Eating Italian: I love Italian food. If you are dining at an Italian restaurant and there are no calorie counts available what should you eat? I find the items that are lowest in calories are raviolis that contain no meat, angel hair pasta with tomatoes and garlic, spaghetti with marinara sauce, thin crust pizza with vegetables. Stay away from any cheese sauces, sausage, meatballs and thick crust pizzas with meats.

Eating Mexican: I like Mexican restaurants. Shrimp or chicken fajitas are low in calories, especially if you don't eat the tortillas. I also get grilled fish and rice entrees. Soft corn tortilla shrimp tacos are a good choice. Stay away from anything fried, large burritos, taquitos, and nachos.

How will I feel?

Let's talk about cravings;

You will have cravings. I would like to tell you this will not happen but it will. I have been on these eating plans for over two years now and I still have cravings. When I go past a Five Guys restaurant I think about having a burger and fries. When I go past Jack in the Box, I think of an Oreo cookie shake. I think about tater tots covered with chili, cheese and onions. I think about a pepperoni pizza with oily cheese dripping from it. Believe me you will have cravings.

I attack the cravings in various ways. If I want something sweet, I eat mandarin oranges, grapes, cantaloupe or watermelon. If I want ice cream I tell myself to get to a eating plan where I can eat the no-sugar-added ice cream. For pizza, I eat vegetarian pizza and only enough slices to meet my calorie limit. You can eat any of your cravings if you keep the calorie count down to whatever eating plan you are following that day, but I know I can't do that with some foods.

I feel hungry: Of course, you are going to feel hungry when you start this eating plan. It's how you respond to this feeling that will determine your success or failure. When you are hungry, snack on some fruit or vegetables without a dip.

Discipline: The commercials on TV of the newest fast food burger or the smell of pizza will make staying on your eating plan difficult. So, what do you do? First you must weigh yourself every day even if you don't want to, even if you cheated the night before. If you weigh yourself, then at least you will know what you are supposed to do. It will make you feel guilty if you decide not to follow the plan. Eventually if you want to lose the weight the guilt will get you back on track. Let's say you get off track, you end up eating a cheeseburger at 10 p.m., you eat half of a large pizza, you can't resist getting an order of chicken wings. It's going to happen and you will enjoy the food. You may feel guilty about what you ate but don't beat yourself up over it. Nobody is perfect. **Continue to weigh yourself every morning**. Stick to the plan and follow the eating guidelines.

Weight plateaus: When I was losing my weight, I would hit weight plateaus where it was more difficult to lose the weight. I am not sure why this occurs. If you seem stuck on a weight just keep on following the eating plans. You will eventually loose the weight.

Summary:

You can change your relationship with food. You have the power! If you start the plan and then get away from it, then simply restart the plan. You will feel better. Start today! There are two additional eating plan examples at the end of the book.

Weight Coach

Weight Coach: If you think you need a weight coach to help you through this process, I am available. Please send me a request at lackman1@aol.com and I will let you know how I can help.

Health Improvement after I lost the weight: My cardiac risk went from dangerous to optimal in a year and a half. Comparing June 2015 to February 2017 my cardiac risk went from 4.67

to 3.06, my overall cholesterol level went from 196 to 157, non-HDL went from 154 to 107, my LDL went from 138 to 93. My triglycerides went from 92 to 38, my HDL (good cholesterol) went from 42 to 52. As stated earlier I am not a doctor and not an expert on the details of what all the above numbers represent but I can tell you that my doctor was impressed with the results.

Let's look at a 10-day example for maintaining desired weight

Day 1:

Carl has been on the eating plans for a year now and he is happy with his weight. He wants to make sure he doesn't gain any weight back. His desired maintenance weight is 180 pounds. Therefore, his weekly goal will always be 180 pounds. He weighs himself Monday morning and he weighs 181 pounds. For today he will follow Eating Plan #2. ***Eating Plan #2 is designed for days where your weight is over your weekly goal by two pounds or less.***

Day 2:

Carl weighs himself Tuesday morning and he weighs 180.5 pounds. His desired maintenance weight is 180 pounds. He is a half a pound above his desired weight. He will follow Eating Plan #2 again today.

Day 3:

Carl weighs himself Wednesday morning. He weighs 179 pounds. His desired maintenance weight is 180 pounds. He is one pound under his goal so he will follow ***Eating Plan # 3 as his weight is at his weekly goal or lower than his goal by two pounds or less.***

Day 4:

Carl weighs himself Thursday morning and he weighs 178.5 pounds. His desired maintenance weight is 180 pounds. Since he is one and a half-pound under his goal he will follow Eating Plan #3 again today.

Day 5:

Carl weighs himself Friday morning and he weighs 177 pounds. His desired maintenance weight is 180 pounds. Since he is three pounds under his goal he will follow ***Eating Plan #4 today as his weight is under his weekly goal between 2.1 to four pounds.***

Day 6:

Carl weighs himself Saturday morning and he weighs 175.5 pounds. His desired maintenance weight is 180 pounds. He is 4.5 pounds under his desired weight. He will follow ***Eating Plan #5 today because his weight is four pounds or more under his goal. He gets to eat anything he wants!***

Day 7:

Carl weighs himself Sunday morning and he weighs 177 pounds. His desired maintenance weight is 180 pounds. Since he is three pounds under his goal he will follow ***Eating Plan #4 today as his weight is under his weekly goal between 2.1 to four pounds.***

Day 8 - New Week:

Carl weighs himself Monday morning and he weighs 179 pounds. This is a new week. He is maintaining his weight now so he does not need to set a new weekly goal. His desired maintenance weight is 180 pounds. He is one pound under his goal so he will follow ***Eating Plan # 3 as his weight is at his weekly goal or lower than his goal by two pounds or less.***

Day 9:

Carl weighs himself Tuesday morning and he weighs 180 pounds. His desired maintenance weight is 180 pounds. He is at his goal. For today he will follow Eating plan #3.

Day 10:

Carl weighs himself Wednesday morning. He weighs 181.2 pounds. His desired maintenance weight is 180 pounds. He is 1.2 pounds above his desired weight. For today he will follow Eating plan #2. ***Eating Plan #2 is designed for days where your weight is over your weekly goal by two pounds or less.***

Continue to follow the eating plans to make sure you maintain your weight!

__Jenny goes on vacation!__

Jenny is heading to beautiful Puerto Vallarta, Mexico. She doesn't want to take a scale with her. The day before she left for vacation she weighed 194 pounds. She is still trying to lose weight. Her weekly goal is 194 pounds. She is at her goal, so during vacation she will follow Eating Plan #3. ***Eating Plan #3 is followed when your weight is at your weekly goal or lower than your goal by two pounds or less.***

Day 1:

Jenny arrives at the airport for an early morning flight. She had an English muffin at home before she left so she wouldn't be tempted by airport food. She takes a three-hour flight, gets through customs, loves her hotel and decides she deserves a few margaritas and a nice lunch. For lunch, she orders grilled Mahi Mahi with rice. For dinner, she can eat what she wants she wants and opts for a burrito. She resists dessert.

Day 2:

For breakfast, she has a fruit cup. The hotel is having a special on fajitas at lunch, so she orders one with grilled chicken and shrimp. She can't resist a banana loco drink which she knows must have many calories. She ends up having two. At dinner, she decides to eat healthier, she orders grilled salmon with broccoli and rice.

Day 3:

Jenny had packed some breakfast bars, so she has one of those in the morning. For lunch, she took a tour which included lunch and tequila tasting. The tequila was great! The lunch on the tour was a taco bar. She had three tacos, two grilled chicken and one pork. She just put veggies, guacamole and salsa on her tacos, no cheese. For dinner, she orders a rib eye steak and she shared a flan.

Day 4:

Jenny had another breakfast bar in the morning. She decided it was time for some more margaritas, she had three. She ordered a grilled chicken salad with balsamic vinegar dressing for lunch. For dinner, she had some fresh caught local tuna with rice.

Day 5:

Jenny had another breakfast bar. The afternoon was spent at the spa snacking on fresh fruit. For dinner, the hotel was throwing a fiesta. There was lots of food. She ate some fresh shrimp, salad, some sushi, and lots of vodka soda and limes.

Day 6:

Jenny slept till noon the next day, too many drinks last night. She ordered some menudo for lunch. For dinner, she ordered a grilled pork chop with fresh vegetables. She had some ice cream for desert. No drinking today.

Day 7:

Jenny had a fruit cup for breakfast. Today she needs to head home. She has lunch at the airport and gets two shrimp tacos. She is home for dinner and has some grilled chicken.

Day 8 - New Week:

Jenny had a great time on vacation. Jenny weighs herself Monday morning and she weighs 195.5 pounds. Since today starts a new week, Jenny has decided to lower her weekly goal by a half a pound this week. Her goal last week was 194 pounds, so her goal this week is now 193.5 pounds. She is two pounds over her weekly goal of 193.5 pounds so today she will follow ***Eating Plan # 2. Eating Plan #2 is designed for days where your weight is over your weekly goal by two pounds or less.***

How To Lose 50 Pounds

<u>Use the table below to help you track your weight and determine your eating plans</u>

<u>My Daily Weight Tracker</u>

Google Doc link for home printing of table: https://tinyurl.com/ya7x9cu3

DATE	Day	What I weighed today	Weekly Weight goal	plus or minus weekly weight goal	Eating plan I will follow today
Eating plans	#1	#2	#3	#4	#5
Your weight today	is more than two pounds over your weekly goal.	is over your weekly goal by two pounds or less	is at your weekly goal or lower than your goal by two pounds or less	is under your weekly goal between 2.1 to four pounds	is four pounds or more under your weekly goal

See eating plan detail page for specific guidelines Notes: Your weekly weight goal changes every seven days until you meet your desired maintenance weight

Dave Lack

Eating plan guide for one page print out

Google Doc link for home printing of table: https://tinyurl.com/y7ulwhsw

Eating plans	Eating Plan #1	Eating Plan #2	Eating Plan #3	Eating Plan #4	Eating Plan #5
Your weight today	is more than two pounds over your weekly goal.	is over your weekly goal by two pounds or less	is at your weekly goal or lower than your goal by two pounds or less	is under your weekly goal between 2.1 to four pounds	is four pounds or more under your weekly goal
Breakfast	200 calories or less	200 calories or less	200 calories or less	one low calorie meal a day, other meals eat what you want	eat what you want
Lunch	350 calories or less	350 calories or less	350 calories or less	one low calorie meal a day, other meals eat what you want	eat what you want
Dinner before 8pm	650 calories or less	900 calories or less	eat what you want	one low calorie meal a day, other meals eat what you want	eat what you want
Dessert	no dessert	no dessert	any dessert under 400 calories	any dessert under 700 calories	eat what you want
Snack	100 calories or less	100 calories or less	100 calories or less	100 calories or less	eat what you want
Vegetables	eat what you want	eat what you want	eat what you want	eat what you want	eat what you want
Fruit	eat what you want	eat what you want	eat what you want	eat what you want	eat what you want

* all dinners in Eating plans one through four must be eaten by 8pm. If after 8 pm dinner, must be under 650 calories. Note # : You may substitute calorie counts between meals. For example if you are in Eating plan two and you want to have a breakfast of 900 calories you can do that but your dinner will need to be 200 calories or less.

In Appreciation

I want to thank my beautiful wife and kids for helping me fine tune my thoughts. I am lucky to be so blessed. I also want to thank my neighbor Matt for providing his input and editing skills.

Dave Lack
<u>Notes</u>

<u>Notes</u>